KETO MEAL PLAN

AN INTRODUCTORY GUIDE TO LIVING THE HEALTHY KETOGENIC LIFESTYLE INCLUDING A 30 DAY WEIGHT LOSS, LOW-CARB, HIGH-FAT, MODERATE-PROTEIN KETO DIET MEAL PLAN

Table of Contents

Chapter 1: Introduction to the Keto Diet

The roots of the Ketogenic or the Keto diet may be difficult to establish clearly. Although this diet may seem like it has only recently been discovered, the first clinical studies which mention the approach was actually as far back as the early 1900's. Interestingly, the diet was first intended to treat epilepsy. In a study published in 1922, Dr. Russell M. Wilder uses what is considered to be one of the first mentions of the terms which are now used with the diet.

Even at that time, the study started from a given basis, like most studies. The foundation of the study was that the Ketogenic diet with its low carbohydrate intake increases the ketone levels in the blood. Ketones are defined as organic compounds which are produced by the body in a state where it is not getting the carbohydrates it needs from foods or in states of starvation. Ketones contain:

- Acetone
- Acetoacetic acid
- Beta-hydroxybutyric acid

These acids are called ketone bodies. The first 1922 study found that these acids increased considerably in the body on the low carbohydrate diet. However, the study has some serious limitations, even if it was charting new territories at its time. The subjects of the study were confined to their beds meaning that their daily caloric needs were reduced. To apply this data to modern day requirements, the caloric expenditure would be considerably higher and even active people who are on the Ketogenic diet would have caloric needs which would be considerably different.

In the 1970s, the Atkins diet made its way as one of the most interesting low-carb plans to lose weight. Researched and published by Dr. Robert C. Atkins, the study was received with mixed opinions. The press at the time noted that most of the ideas of Dr. Atkins were actually rejected by the medical community. But even so, the Ketogenic diet has become very popular again, especially with people who are into fitness and who hope to lower their body fat percentage levels with this approach.

The Evolutionary Perspective

Before the studies of the 1900's, the Ketogenic diet principles were still present, but maybe in different forms and in different places around the world. One such place was Greenland, at least until recently; this isolated island had little food variation. Largely based on seafood, fish, mussels or shrimp, the Greenlandic diet is here to show that a different approach to carbohydrate consumption is not necessarily new. Based on a diet which mainly consisted of protein and fats, the Greenlandic diet is one of the many examples of the sustainability which can come from foods which are low in carbs.

In other places around the world, the access to carbohydrates was not as restricted. Even so, the changing of the seasons also impacted the nutrition of people meaning that carbohydrate consumption was largely diminished during winter time and colder months of the year.

Some studies even cite early experiments with fasting and alternating diets as soon as 400 BC in ancient Greece. Using different types of food and water restrictions, these diets were often used for the treatment of various diseases, which include epilepsy.

It can be said that the principles of food alternation and various levels of restriction were not new when they came to life in the early 1900's studies. But at the same time, this practice started to fade away with the appearance of seizure medication. In some cases, this medication would not be successful. Many of these experiments and studies were carried out on periods between 18 to 25 days and they included severe caloric restrictions. There are a main number of ideas which can be drawn from this spectacular history of the Keto diet:

- Lower caloric intake
- Adjacent health benefits
- Diet duration

The lower caloric intake is one of the main points of discussion with the Keto diet. Although its primary role was to treat seizures and epilepsy, the diet was strongly rooted in a lower calorie intake. Thus, if you plan to lose weight yourself with the diet, you need to be prepared to reduce daily calories as well.

Modern studies show that one of the few diets which actually shows cognition benefits comes with fasting. In combination with a lower carbohydrate intake, fasting might have been one of the first triggers of improved brain health. It can be said that if you also plan to see improved cognition, you might want to consider the options you have with fasting which refers to the periods in which you do not consume any calories at all.

Chapter 2: Keto Diet Purposes

The Keto diet's resurgence in popularity is based on many historical facts. At the same time, there is plenty of misinformation when it comes to what this diet should actually look like. Stripping it from all advice which can complicate it for the average dieter, the Keto diet can be simplified considerably.

Basically, the Ketogenic diet represents a very low-carb and very high-fat diet. In figures, this looks surprising for many people, but the maximum carbohydrate daily intake percentage is at 5%. The diet can be simplified as follows:

- 5% carbohydrate intake
- 20% protein intake
- 75% fats intake

These percentages represent parts of the total daily 100% caloric intake. For most people, this means that they can consume up to 50 grams of carbohydrates every day while on the Ketogenic diet. Even more, these carbohydrates are also largely consumed indirectly from foods such as vegetables which are high in fiber. This is why people on the Ketogenic diet will not typically consume other types of carbs such as bread or pastries.

The Purposes of the Keto Diet

With these figures in mind, people tend to believe that the Keto diet is a plausible solution for fat loss. This is mainly triggered by two theories which are yet to be fully proven in their claims.

a) The first theory is based on insulin production. The idea is to keep insulin levels low during the Keto diet. Since insulin is also responsible for Lipogenesis, it is believed that severely restricting carbohydrate consumption will lead to a better mobilization of fats. In other words, people believe that influencing insulin production can lead to fat loss. In certain cases, they believe this to be the solution to fat loss plateaus. These periods refer to the stages in which people see no progress with their weight loss process.

b) The second theory is based on an advantage of the Ketogenic diet over other low carbohydrate diets. Based on the idea that the body requires more energy and more effort to convert proteins to glucose, the theory claims that the body works extra hard for this purpose. In turn, this would mean it burns more body fat to achieve this goal.

These theories can have some reasoning behind them but their critique is strong as well. Often seen as simplistic, the first theory implies that insulin is controlled by carbohydrates. But this is only partially true. Protein can also be insulinogenic. What this means is that you can also store fat and gain weight while consuming zero carbohydrates. This is due to the ASD (Acylation Stimulating Protein) hormone.

The second theory has also been received with mixed opinions. There are a limited number of studies which actually show that there is no direct benefit when it comes to weight loss when you use fat and protein for energy. But at the same time, this theory can have some grounding in the idea that it can suppress appetite.

It has been shown that controlling carbohydrate intake can control appetite as well. At the same time, the slower digestive process which usually comes with fats and proteins will also help you stay fuller for longer periods of time.

The Advantages of the Keto Diet

While the diet has no unique advantage over similar caloric plans, it does stand out from the crowd when it comes to reducing appetite and eliminating foods. In turn, this leads to a diet which is basically a form of reducing daily calories.

Appetite Control

Controlling appetite can be difficult to achieve. For many people, this involves strong motivation and the required dedication to maintain it over a sufficient period of time in order to see weight loss results. While the Keto diet might not be the best way of controlling appetite, its aggressive plan can carry some people over certain periods of stagnation in weight loss which is also referred as a plateau in the fitness community.

Food Elimination

When it comes to eliminating carbohydrates, this step can also be limiting solution. This is why it can actually be detrimental over longer periods of time as well. While there are better solutions when it comes to reducing calories while still consuming a balanced diet, this advantage can also be seen as a great benefit for those who are struggling to see any results with other weight loss plans. It can also be described as aggressive by some people and this is why the Keto diet is not the easiest diet to follow.

The Proven Benefits of the Keto Diet

When it comes to data which supports the Keto diet and similar restrictive meal plans, there is sufficient evidence to sustain their results. This can be true, at least for a number of people on the diet. The idea is backed by a 2014 meta-analysis which looked at multiple studies and diets similar to or which included the Keto diet. During the analysis, it was realized that the Keto diet does come with positive benefits and that it also does this in a short period of time. Unfortunately, this is where most analyzed cases stopped showing improvements for longer periods of time as the lower weight was hard to maintain after the diet.

As a person who is trying to lose weight with the Ketogenic diet, you need to know that what you do once the diet is over is crucially important to keep your new lower weight. Statistically speaking, most people fail at this task so please read more on how to maintain dieting results later on in this book.

A 2013 meta-analysis published in the *Journal of Nutrition* looked at specific studies which only targeted the Keto approach with its limited carbohydrate consumption to 50 grams per day. Most of the 13 studies carried out found that people lost an average of 1kg on the Keto diet. But at the same time, the analysis also notes that this might not be too representative in some cases as the diet is hard to maintain over a longer period of time to see more significant results.

It is also true that many of these benefits can actually be attributed to other nutritional changes as well. One of the changes can be represented by higher protein intake. If you start to consume protein which is more thermogenic than carbs, you will also need more energy to fully metabolize it. Interestingly, protein is also more satiating when compared to other macronutrients.

This, in turn, can lead to the consumption of a lower number of calories to the satiating feel which comes with higher protein consumption. But over long periods of time, things begin to equalize if you consume more protein to balance the lower carbs intake. Furthermore, protein plays a crucial role when it comes to maintaining muscle mass as well, which is also responsible for better fat loss success.

In this case, you are facing a strict pre-diet and post-diet plan, as a well-executed Keto diet can produce results in terms of weight loss. You also have to remember that the body is highly adaptive and it will not respond in the same way with other diets you might plan after your first Keto diet.

Chapter 3: How to Prepare For the Keto Diet?

While the specific benefits of the Keto diet are not as compelling as many people expect, you may still want to try it yourself, especially under a stricter approach. This is where it is important to note that there are some small preparation steps you can take when looking to maximize your success with the diet.

Preparing for the foods you are about to consume is key. The planning stage can make or break the diet and this is why you need to prepare in advance. The first thing you need to anticipate is the elimination of the carbohydrates from your diet.

Consider Lowering Carbohydrates

Since it can be brutal to adapt to the diet in the first few weeks, you can experiment the low-carbohydrate approach for an entire day before deciding to go on the diet. The Ketogenic diet is very strict when it comes to the nutrients you can consume and to those which you exclude. Since you are going to exclude all grains and their nutrients, you can even begin to do this on certain days before the diet, not because of the weight loss benefits but to better establish the types of foods you can source and the types of meals you can prepare.

While most foods which are recommended on the Ketogenic diet are actually easily available in most supermarkets, you also need to consider their overall cost and quality as well. But most importantly, you need to see if they are actually sustainable for your daily meals with your own lifestyle. Some things to consider include:

The Time Needed To Prepare Meals

Some meals take longer to prepare than others. If you have a busy schedule and especially if you have a family to look after, you need to realize that you will need to prepare separate meals for yourself. This involves more time in the kitchen and in many cases, preparing the meals in advanced can be the only option if you want to save time.

Meals You Can Consume At Work

While away from home, you can find that sticking to the diet can be more challenging. This is where you might be tempted by various quick snacks which are often very high in carbohydrates. The best solution is to prepare your meals in advance and take them with you to work. If this is not possible, you should always have a Keto supplement on hand to provide your body the nutrition it needs during this otherwise stressful period.

Resting Time

As one of the areas which often get overlooked before planning the Keto diet, resting is crucial. You need to get enough sleep every night, especially during the first and the second week of the diet when your body begins to adapt to the dietary changes. In some cases, people are fine with only 6 hours of sleep every night but since you might feel more tired while on the Keto diet, you might need to get at least 8 hours of sleep every night. To make this achievable, you will need to go to bed early or even switch off electronics such as the TV or phone before going to bed in order to fall asleep faster.

Workouts and Physical Activity

If you plan to stay active on the diet, you can expect a drop in performance which can come in various forms. It is here that you can expect to lift lighter weights if you train at the gym. But you can also expect lower endurance if you are a fan of cardiovascular workouts. You need to plan your exercises accordingly with shorter workouts. At the same time, you can consider the supplements which are made specifically for this goal and the active people on the Keto diet.

Alcohol Consumption

Generally speaking, alcohol consumption is not right for the Keto diet or for your health in general. Reducing the amount of consumed alcohol or even eliminating it is highly advised. If you do not want to see drops in energy levels or further dizziness during the first week on the diet, you should stay away from alcohol. From the strict carbohydrates perspective, the amount you get from alcohol is insignificant. For example, there is only up to 4 grams of carbs per bottle of beer.

Set a Budget and Improve Savings

Setting a budget for the Keto diet is highly advisable. The foods you consume within 30 days are not cheap and you may even want to add some supplements to achieve the best results. Simply calculating a daily budget for foods is recommended.

The price should not be the only variable to consider when it comes to making better choices. Food quality is also important. Fresh produce is crucial and you can do all you can to get these types of foods. A good idea is to look at the foods you can source from your local farmers market. In many cases, you can find great foods like meats and eggs which are even healthier than the options you find in supermarkets. At the same time, you also have the ability to find fresh seasonal foods at a farmers market. Therefore, instead of consuming frozen foods with not much nutritional value, you can focus on fresh ingredients which are always recommended for weight loss.

Buy In Bulk

Bulk buying is one of the best tips you can apply when preparing for the Keto diet. Many foods can be cheaper this way and you can start with the basics and make your way up to the least essential foods. This is where it is worth considering the options you have at your local supermarkets. Many of these shops have new offers every week so it is worth seeing what is on sale on your particular dieting week.

Plan Fats Intake

Fats represent the most important macronutrient on the Ketogenic diet. With 75% of the total daily nutritional intake, fats need to be planned before you actually start the diet. At the very least, you should know where to buy the fats you need when you begin the diet. Saturated fats, monosaturated fats and polyunsaturated fats such as Omega 3 are recommended on the Keto diet.

Consider MCT Oil

As one of the leading sources of healthy fats, MCT oil represents a complex solution which is often seen as a starter for the modern Keto diet. Medium Chain Triglycerides or MCT oil represents one of the best options when it comes to fatty acids intake.

But not all MCT oils are the same and this is why you need to know that there are many other subtypes of oils which can even be purchased separately for the Keto diet. While all oils derived from coconuts are generally regarded as healthy, not all of them are actually able to offer the weight loss trigger you need. Many MCT oils are rich in Lauric acid, which might be healthy but they are not the best option derived from coconuts for weight loss. MCT oil is formed from:

Caproic Acid – C6

Caproic Acid or C6 is one of the acids found in coconut oil. It converts into ketones really fast but it comes in small concentrations in coconut oil. The oil is easy to identify as it comes with a bad taste and an unpleasant smell. If your MCT oil comes with a weird aftertaste or causes you to have stomach issues, this might be due to the fact the C6 oil wasn't properly removed in the distillation process.

Caprylic Acid – C8

Caprylic Acid, known as C8 or *Brain Octane* oil is one of the most qualitative oils to consider for your Ketogenic diet. It comes with a high concentration of C8 acid which means that manufacturers need 18 tablespoons of coconut oil to produce one tablespoon of Caprylic acid. Since the acid doesn't need to be processed by the liver, it is fast to absorb and this makes it crucial for those on the Ketogenic diet. At the same time, *Brain Octane* comes with good gut benefits and brain benefits as well.

With its antimicrobial action, it is one of the foods to consider for fast results on the Keto diet. You can consume it plainly or you can also consume it mixed in certain drinks such as coffee or green tea. As a general preparation tip, you should be aware that the oil will change the texture of these drinks I recommend that you try the mix before you start the diet. Used for the *Bulletproof coffee*, the acid can come with impressive cognition benefits. Because it requires high amounts of coconut oil to produce, it is one of most expensive types of acids to be consumed during the Ketogenic diet.

Lauric Acid – C12

Lauric acid needs to be processed by the liver as it contains 50% of coconut oil. This means that, technically, it is not a medium chain triglyceride but rather a long chain triglyceride as it doesn't absorb as fast as the other MCT's. It can also come with antimicrobial action but it may not be as effective as the other options. The oil is acceptable, but if you want the best solutions, the C6, C8, and C19 prove to be better options.

Other Types of Acids

Acids C14 and above are rarer to find in a pure form. But they are widely used in other foods and supplements such as meal replacements you can encounter while on the diet. The C18 group is widely available in these supplements. The three acids forming C18 include linoleic acid, oleic acid, and stearic acid. Mostly saturated, these acids also have to be processed by the liver.

Combinations of oils are also available. While the C8 Brain Octane is often found on its own, XCT oil combines C8 and C10 acids. So when you plan to enter the Keto diet, you need to know that these oils can even be used at different times of the day when you want to see their benefits:

Brain Octane or the C8 acid, in its purest form, is to be consumed in the morning with coffee as it comes with the most benefits in terms of cognition. XCT oil which combines C8 and C10 acids are more affordable but are slower to digest. This is why it can be consumed through the day for its brain benefits and to help the fat burn process.

Cold-Pressed Coconut Oil for Added Fats

Cold-pressed oil can be one of the more affordable alternatives to MCT oil. Its name comes from its extraction technique. The oil is mechanically extracted from coconuts at low temperatures. This means that it maintains its nutritional value better and when you take into consideration that it is actually not refined or processed further, it comes as one of the most valuable options for healthy fats intake on the Keto diet.

Coconut oil is also widely available in most supermarkets and it comes with information on the calories per 100ml or less as well. In comparison to olive oil, it has been proven to be superior in quality as the medium chain triglycerides are faster to absorb than the long-chain triglycerides. In essence, it also comes with some of the benefits of the above MCT oil which also include cardiovascular benefits with increased HDL Cholesterol levels and with an antimicrobial action as well.

Palm Fruit Oil

Another interesting alternative is palm fruit oil. Although not as available as coconut oil, it comes with proven benefits for better fats intake. The oleic fruit is turned into oil and it delivers 50% saturated fats, 40% unsaturated fats and 10% polyunsaturated fats. This makes it a complex solution which is not as fast to absorb as MCT oil but can be represented as a viable alternative. The saturated fats of the oil also make it a practical option when it comes to cooking. The oil is safer for cooking at higher temperatures when compared to similar cooking oils and it can be one of the additions to your Ketogenic diet.

The palm fruit oil also comes with a series of benefits which can be recommended for further health improvements. It manages to fight free radicals and also protects the heart with its flavonoids. The oil has also been researched due to its water-soluble micronutrients such as Vitamin E which can also prove beneficial for cardiovascular health.

Olive Oil

One of the most widely available alternatives is olive oil. Virgin olive oil comes with 73% saturated fats, Omega 3, Omega 6, Vitamin E and Vitamin K. Virgin olive oil also contains active antioxidants. As one of the oils which can also be consumed post-diet, it comes with a series of potential health benefits which can be recommended in many situations.

The antioxidants in the virgin olive oil can have a role in decreasing or keeping inflammation away. It also has benefits for Arthritis, Alzheimer's and other heart diseases. While it can be used for various cooking recipes, olive oil can also represent one of the options to consume raw to maintain the fatty acids molecule bonds. Some shops also store fresh olive oils which can also represent as a great alternative.

Flaxseed

Flaxseed is also widely available in stores as many of its benefits are similar to the oils above, it is also worth noting that studies show it to be a good solution for constipation or diarrhea, which can occur in some ketosis cases. The oil is also a viable option for weight loss results as it has been shown to increase collagen production. Collagen is one of the proteins which can improve the natural look and elasticity of the skin. When you are trying to lose weight, regaining your skin's elasticity is crucial and this is why adding it to your Ketogenic meal plan can be a great solution for better weight loss results.

Macadamia Nuts

As one of the tastiest sources of healthy fats, macadamia nuts are a great addition to your ketogenic diet. Like many similar products, you will have to watch their calories as you can easily max out your daily target. With 718 calories per 100 grams, it represents one of the most caloric foods to be recommended for the Ketogenic diet. But at the same time, the same quantity comes with 76 grams of fats. Consumed in various forms, macadamia nuts also come with a rich content of Magnesium, Vitamin B-6, Iron, and Calcium.

But is this important? You can experience some issues adapting to the Keto diet and one way this problem manifests itself is with dizziness. This is why it is important to consider the minerals in the calorie-rich macadamia nuts as a great tool for better overall health during this stressful period. If you are an active person, macadamia nuts can also represent a great snack full of minerals and of healthy fats to be consumed before workouts.

Avocado

As one of the foods which you may already know, avocado represents a great source of healthy fats. It comes with an increased satiety and a higher calorie count which can be recommended for active people. With 15 grams of fat per 100 grams, avocado comes with 20% of your daily folate needs as well. This makes it a viable option when it comes to overall health benefits and when you consider its positive impact on brain and mood, avocado also represents one of the foods you can continue consuming long after your diet is completed.

Studies show that the versatile avocado also plays a positive role when it comes to the digestion of the nutrients which come from plants. But most importantly, avocado increases satiety. It can therefore be used in various scenarios in which you might feel hungry during the Keto diet.

Butter

Butter can also be a versatile solution used for cooking as well. It is unlike any other food as it comes with 81 grams of fat per 100 grams. Grass-fed butter is clearly the leading choice and with only 0.1 grams of carbohydrates, butter represents a viable solution for fats intake. With short chain and medium chain fatty acids, grass-fed butter is rich in Vitamin A. This vitamin is important when it comes to the health of your skin and even for the mucous membranes.

Butter comes with a combination of short chain and medium chain triglycerides (MCT) which are immediately converted into energy. Instead of your body storing the fats from butter, it actually turns into energy with a very fast action. This makes butter and products derived from coconut oil a worthwhile option when it comes to pre-workout foods and snacks. You can also add butter to various foods and proteins which can come as a more simple way of consuming it.

Chicken and Duck Fat

Chicken fat can also come with a good complexity which mixes faster and slower digestion of fats. With 30 grams of saturated fats, 21 grams of polyunsaturated fats and 45 grams of monosaturated fats per 100 grams, chicken fat can also add flavor to your otherwise restricted foods during the ketogenic diet.

Protein

Protein is one of the most important macronutrients of the ketogenic diet. It helps to meet your caloric needs with a complexity which protects your body from muscle loss in this stressing period. At the same time, protein plays a vital role in brain health as well.

One of the most important benefits of protein is achieving muscular health. Protein is essential for muscle growth and at the same time, it can also be responsible for maintaining your muscle mass over a period of 30 days where your diet sees important changes.

There are various sources of animal and plant-based proteins and the leading options should always be explored when it comes to the Ketogenic diet. Based on various amino acids which are the building blocks of protein, this macronutrient is important for the better overall sustainability of your muscles, immune system, and nervous system. At the same time, protein can also be used for energy but you want to avoid this by following the overall percentages which are recommended when it comes to macronutrient intake during the diet. All proteins are based on amino acids which are also categorized as follows:

Essential Amino Acids

These amino acids cannot be synthesized by the body and you will need to get them from foods. The 9 amino acids include isoleucine, leucine, histidine, methionine, lycine, phenylalanine, threonine, tryptophan, and valine.

Non-Essential Amino Acids

These amino acids are usually made by the body from protein digestion. The amino acids include asparagine, alanine, aspartic and glutamic acid.

Conditional Amino Acids

Conditional amino acids have an interesting role. They are used by the body during stress, sickness or for better nutrient transport. They include arginine, glutamine, cysteine, glycine, ornithine, proline, tyrosine and serine.

These amino acids are present in different quantities in the products you consume regularly or on the diet. Most of them can also be isolated or formulated in different supplements. One way you will see them listed specifically like this is with amino acid drinks, which can be highly recommended on the Ketogenic diet. There are different types of protein and they can be rotated every day to have a more enjoyable diet.

Nuts and Seeds

Nuts and seeds are widely available and are a very handy snack to have in your store cupboard. They can be consumed before workouts, after workouts, in salad and at any time of the day. Rich in protein and minerals, nuts and seeds represent a small but healthy snack. Their unique mineral content can help to prevent certain problems which can arise for active people such as muscle cramps.

Coconut milk

Coconut milk contains a small amount of protein but it represents an opportunity when it comes to its high-fat content as well. With up to 24 grams of fat per 100 grams of milk, it represents one of the delicious drinks you can consume during the diet. Since it is also high in fats, it can be one of the drinks to consider early in the morning to boost your overall energy levels. With better availability over recent years, it is an alternative which is also more affordable than it used to be.

Whey

As the most popular type of protein in supplements, whey protein deserves its place among the top protein sources on the ketogenic diet. The micronized form of whey which is present in supplements such as meal replacements or protein shakes makes it one of the proteins with a complete chain of amino acids which is also fast to digest.

This makes it a practical option when it comes to better overall nutrition before the workout, after a workout or as needed through the day. The good news is that the thousands of whey products which are available on the market are also made with great flavor profiles which can be derived from natural sources as well.

There are different types of whey protein as well. Grass-fed options are the clear winner if you are looking for pure quality. But you can also find concentrated whey as well as isolate whey. The concentrated formulation comes with around 80% protein content while isolate whey contains over 90% protein content. Free from carbohydrates, isolate protein is an effective solution if you want to improve weight loss results.

By itself, the whey protein shakes might not be as filling as you'd hope and this is why they are often consumed with a meal as well. Their advantage is practicality and this is where it manages to offer you a protein boost even when you are away from home.

Organ Meats

Meats such as liver, heart, kidneys, sweetbreads, brain, tongue or tripe represent a great protein source as well. The liver is considered to be the best source for nutrient complexity. At the same time, it represents a meat which also comes with Vitamin A which is great for our eyes and with Vitamin B and D. Liver also contains iron, phosphorus, copper, and magnesium which are all recommended for strength and immunity during the ketogenic diet.

Eggs

As one of the complete and affordable sources of protein, eggs represent a practical option. You can consume eggs early in the morning for a boost of fats and protein. You can also consume eggs as needed to meet your caloric goals if you feel your ketosis is not going according to plan since it is always easy to boil them and serve them immediately.

Poultry

Chicken is one of the most consumed sources of protein for weight loss around the world. It is not specific to Ketogenic weight loss but its high quantity of protein and low quantity of carbohydrates recommends it when it comes to better overall nutrient availability. It also acts to protect muscle loss and it can aid you in your scope of reducing body fat percentages.

Grass-fed Meat

Grass-fed meats such as beef represent a slower-digesting protein. It can be one of the proteins to be consumed at lunch or at dinner since it takes longer to digest. As a result, it feeds your muscles through the night and it allows your muscles to recover better, especially in the conditions in which you cannot count on carbohydrates to do this.

There are different types of beef options to consider. Grass-fed beef is the best solution at the moment, even if it doesn't represent the most affordable option.

Fish

Fish is high in fats and protein and this makes it one of the leading foods to be consumed on the Ketogenic diet. If you want the best fats, salmon is one of the great options to consider for all types of meals. Trout also represents one of the high-quality sources of protein and it can be the foundation of a great meal on the diet. Other types of sea fish can also be considered. Seafood is also one of the great options but you will need to consider the choices you have when it comes to better overall budgeting since it might not be the most affordable food.

Chapter 4: Meal Plan

Before you start cooking, it is important to know that you are eating for function and not so much for pleasure during the diet. The aim is to simplify the meals as much as possible as this gives you the ability to actually stay on the diet. The last thing you want is to start cooking complicated foods which take time and which push you further from your caloric goal.

There are thousands of recipes to consider and noting some of them is a good way to start. In order to simplify them even further, dividing the meals into breakfast, lunch, dinner and meal replacements are the best way to go. Over the duration of 30 days or four weeks, you can choose to consume different combinations of the following meals. They are not as high in calories as you might expect and this is due to their high fats content which is very satiating. At the same time, all the meals can be used in a

combination with the recommended Keto
supplements which are also based on fats and
protein.

Ketogenic Diet Breakfast Meals

There are different ways breakfast is seen on the Keto diet. It can be consumed with a different approach every day, with the same approach every day or you can even skip breakfast altogether. *Bulletproof coffee* can be an alternative.

Bulletproof Coffee

As one of the staple drinks of the Ketogenic diet, *Bulletproof coffee* is one of the best options to start your day. Often consumed by those who are also fasting early in the morning the coffee is easy to make. You will need:

- 1 Cup of Coffee
- 1 Tablespoon of MCT Oil
- 1 Tablespoon of Grass-Fed Unsalted Butter

Fat - 18.2g | Protein 1g | Carbohydrates - 4g | Calories – 158

You can blend the black coffee together with the other two ingredients. In case you want to boost your fats intake, you can also double the quantities of MCT oil and butter. Please note that this will considerably change the texture of the coffee, making it creamier and also harder to consume for some people. As a way to start your Keto diet days, it can be hard to match in terms of energy sources.

There are plenty of great options to consider if you want to have something to eat for breakfast as well. Not all of them are as fast to prepare but having a few options to consider or even abiding by a single breakfast meal for the entire duration of the diet can be an option. This is up to you.

Breakfast No.1 – Fried Eggs with Vegetables and Bacon

Fried eggs are one of the favorite breakfast meals for many people. For this breakfast you have two protein sources coming from eggs and bacon but you also have the added vegetables for micronutrient intake as well. You will need:

- 2 Large Eggs
- 2 Pieces of Sliced Bacon
- 1 Tablespoon of Olive Oil
- ½ Cup of Mushrooms
- ¾ Cups of Spinach

Fats – 30.03g | Protein – 18.7g | Carbs – 2.9g | Calories - 320

This breakfast can be prepared fresh every morning. As an alternate solution, you can change the olive oil to other types of oil if you want to vary fats as well.

You need to place the olive oil on a nonstick pan first. Alternatively, you can also use an olive oil spray to glaze the pan when needed. The pieces of bacon can be lightly fried on each side. When done, they can be removed and placed on a clean plate.

You can now add the spinach and mushrooms. They need to cook until wilted. The spinach and mushrooms can also be placed on the plate next to the bacon. For the final step, you will fry the two eggs so that the yolks remain runny. Place the eggs on top of the spinach and mushrooms for serving.

Breakfast No.2 – Scrambled Eggs

A simpler breakfast can involve just eggs and butter. This option is a good solution during a busy morning when you do not have the time to sauté vegetables. To prepare the breakfast, you will need:

- 2 Whole Eggs
- 1oz. Butter
- Salt and Pepper

Fats – 15.5g | Protein – 14.9g | Carbs – 0.8g| Calories – 259

This breakfast is easy to prepare and the only way you can go wrong with it is by actually allowing the melting butter to turn brown before adding the eggs.

To prepare the breakfast, you need to beat the eggs in a bowl until blended. You will then melt the butter in a nonstick pan. The eggs are always added gently and pulled with a spatula across the pan. The eggs are cooked when there is no more liquid and they become thickened. Finally, you can add salt and pepper before serving.

Breakfast No.3 – Cheese with Sausages

Sausages are also popular for breakfast in some parts of the world. If you want a change from eggs, you can prepare a high-protein and high-fat breakfast with sausages. You will need:

- 1 Sausage
- 1 Cup of Bell Peppers
- 1 Tablespoon of Olive Oil
- 1oz of Cheese

Fats – 31g | Protein – 21g | Carbs – 8g | Calories - 393

Preparing this breakfast is not complicated and you can even add roasted bell peppers if you prepare them in advance and keep them in the fridge to be used as needed.

Using regular or spray olive oil, you can glaze a pan as needed. The sausage is fried evenly on each side. Before it is done, you need to add the chopped bell peppers to the pan as well. After a couple of minutes, you remove the sausage and peppers from the pan placing them on a clean plate. The cheese is freshly grated on top before serving.

Breakfast No.4 – Cheese Roll-Ups

This simple low-calorie breakfast can be an alternative when you do not feel like eating a more complex meal or when you plan to have some type of physical activity like going to the gym in the morning. Avoiding training on an empty stomach is easy with the cheese roll-ups. To prepare them, you will need:

- 8oz. Cheddar
- 2oz. Butter

Fats – 19.6g | Protein - 6.8g | Carbs – 0.4g | Calories - 1020

You will need to spread the butter on the cheese slices using a knife. You need to add butter to each slice of cheese. If your butter does not easily spread, you can consider keeping it outside the fridge before for an hour bore use. After the butter is spread, you will roll-up every slice by hand. Alternatively, you can look for other types of cheese to use, such as provolone.

Breakfast No.5 – BHB Ketones Shake

Beta hydroxy-butyrate (BHB) supplements are now available for many people. They come with zero carbs or sugars and they can instantly raise ketone levels in the body. To prepare this simple shake you will need:

- 1 Scoop of BHB Ketones
- 10 Ounces of Water

Fats – 0 | Protein – 0 | Carbs – 0 | Calories - 15

The shake can be consumed early in the morning but it can also be consumed before a workout if you are the person playing a sport or if you are about to train at your local gym.

Breakfast No.6 – Keto Porridge

Porridge can also be highly Keto-friendly. It comes to meet your needs on the days you have time to prepare a breakfast over the stove. To prepare this delicious breakfast you will need to following ingredients:

- 1oz. Coconut Oil
- 1 Egg
- 1 Tablespoon of Coconut Flour
- 1 Pinch of Cinnamon
- 4 Tablespoons of Coconut Cream

Fats – 62.8g | Protein - 14.3g | Carbs – 19.4g | Calories – 712

To prepare the porridge, you will need to slowly mix the ingredients in a pan. With a low heat, you stir to your liking until you have the texture you enjoy the most. This breakfast is typically served with coconut milk. Fresh or frozen berries can also be added to top the porridge.

Breakfast No.7 – Keto Latte

If you want a drink which is more consistent than *Bulletproof coffee* but you also want to stay away from supplements, a Keto latte can be a delicious alternative. To prepare this unique drink you will need the following ingredients:

- 2 Eggs
- 2 Tablespoons of Coconut Oil
- 1 Cup Of Boiling Water
- 1 Teaspoon of Ground Ginger
- 2 Drops of Vanilla Extract
- 1 Teaspoon of Instant Coffee

Fats – 23.6g | Protein – 6.8g | Carbs – 1g | Calories - 278

These ingredients need to be blended together. You start by boiling water. The coconut oil is placed in a cup where you mix it with a little bit of boiled water. You then add the eggs to the cup as well, blending them with a hand-held blender.

The instant coffee is mixed separately with boiled water in a cup. When it is mixed well, you add it to the coconut oil and eggs together with the vanilla and ginger. All the ingredients are blended together at the end. The drink is best while warm and it is not recommended to be consumed before it gets cold.

Ketogenic Diet Lunch Meals

Lunch can be an important meal on the Ketogenic diet. It marks the second or even the first meal in some cases and this is why it is worth making it with fresh ingredients. In many cases, lunch needs to be prepared in advance. If you are at work, the best solution is to simply pack your lunch with you to avoid the cravings for unhealthy meals at work.

Lunch No.1 – BLT Lettuce Wrap

This traditional lunch idea can be reinvented for the diet. But instead of the classic wrap, you will use bacon. The best part is that this wrap can be done with many ingredients. You can start with the following options:

- 6 Pieces of Bacon
- 2oz. Grilled Chicken
- 1oz. Cheese

- 3 Leaves of Lettuce
- 3 Tablespoons of Mayonnaise

Fats – 39g | Protein – 36g | Carbs – 3.5g | Calories - 425

To prepare the wraps you will need to cook the bacon thoroughly on each side. The same is done with the finely-sliced chicken which needs to be grilled in a pan. To make the wraps, you will lay each slide of bacon separately. On top of the bacon, you will add the slices chicken which is followed by half of the lettuce leaf. The lettuce is topped with mayonnaise and grated cheese. Other vegetables are often used as well in the wrap including sliced tomatoes or sliced pickles. At the end, each slice is rolled with its ingredients to be served as a wrap.

Lunch No.2 – Beef and Avocado Salad

This simple and healthy salad can be a filling option for the diet. With plenty of protein and high in fats, it represents a possible solution for a quick lunch idea. You will need the following:

- 3oz. Ground Beef
- 2 Tablespoons of Chili Seasoning
- 3 Cherry Tomatoes
- ¼ Avocado
- 2 Cups of Lettuce

Fats – 24.3g | Protein – 19g | Carbs – 9g | Calories – 110

To make the salad, you will first need to prepare the ground beef. Using a nonstick pan, you will add the beef gradually stirring and mixing it on all sides until cooked. When done, you will start preparing the rest of the ingredients. The cherry tomatoes will be sliced into thin pieces using a chef's knife. The avocado also needs to be sliced thinly. The lettuce will be chopped in larger pieces and added to a bowl. All the ingredients are now ready to be mixed together.

If you want to slightly increase fats, you will lightly spray some olive oil on the ingredients before mixing them together and adding the chili seasoning. The simple salad can often be made with other ingredients. You can always change the seasoning but keep in mind that chili is thermogenic and recommended for weight loss.

Lunch No.3 – Smoked Salmon with Fresh Spinach

The simple plate of smoked salmon with fresh spinach is one of the Keto-friendly options you can consume fresh every day. Its preparation only takes a couple of minutes and can be done even at work. The ingredients you need include:

- 3/4lb of Smoked Salmon
- 2oz. Spinach
- 1 Tablespoon of Olive Oil
- 1 Lime
- Salt and Pepper

Fats – 31.6g | Protein – 33.9g | Carbs – 3.1g | Calories - 426

This simple lunch is easy to prepare. First, the sliced smoked salmon is placed on a plate. In a bowl, you will mix the fresh spinach with the olive oil. When done, you will plate the spinach next to the salmon. Salt and pepper are added to both the spinach and the salmon. The lime is sliced into two pieces.

Before serving, you will squeeze the lime on top of the salmon. Alternatively, you can also use mayonnaise with this plate as well. In most cases, it can also be a meal you can also consume long after your diet is over as a healthy option.

Lunch No.4 – Quesadillas

This delicious meal with a Keto spin can represent one of the more complex meals of the diet. But its nutrients are perfect and go hand in hand with your macronutrient targets as well. Here is what you will need:

- 2 Eggs and 2 Egg Whites
- 6oz. Cream Cheese
- 1 Tablespoon of Coconut Flour
- ½ Tablespoon of Psyllium
- ½ Teaspoon Salt

Fats – 43.6g|Protein – 14.8g|Carbs – 24.5g|Calories – 884

You first need to beat the whole eggs and the egg whites using a mixer. When you reach a fluffy texture you can add the cream cheese mixing the eggs until you reach a smooth texture. The coconut flour is mixed separately with the psyllium and salt. Following this, you will need to combine all ingredients together while beating.

Before placing the mixture in the oven, please allow it to sit for a few minutes. On a baking sheet, you can spread the mixture well in a square shape with a spatula. You then place it in a preheated oven at 400 degrees Fahrenheit (200 degrees Celsius). After 5-7 minutes, the mix will begin to turn brown on the edges as a sign it is done. Alternatively, you can fry the mixture similarly to pancakes for a rounded shape which is closer to traditional quesadillas.

Lunch No.5 - Keto Caesar Salad

Caesar salad is one of the most popular options for a tasty and lightweight lunch. You can also prepare a Keto version which is simplified but which still abides by the principles of the diet. You will need:

- 2lbs Chicken Breast
- 1 Tablespoon of Olive Oil
- 1 Romaine Lettuce
- 2oz Grated Parmesan
- 1 Tablespoon of Dijon and Lemon Zest

Fats – 28.6g | Protein – 54.8g | Carbs – 4g | Calories – 553

To prepare the simple salad, you will need to grill the chicken first. After the meat is ready, you can cut it into thin pieces to prepare it for the salad. The lettuce is chopped into larger strips. Using a large bowl, you can add the lettuce and the chicken.

You can now add the Dijon mustard and the zest of a lemon according to preference together with seasoning. You need to ensure you mix the ingredients well before serving.

Lunch No.6 – Tuna Avocado Salad

As one of the best sources of fats, avocado is versatile in the kitchen. Combined with tuna, it also comes with increased protein per serving as well. Low in carbohydrates, the salad is easy to make.

- 1 Can of Tuna
- ½ Avocado
- 1 Egg
- 2 Tablespoons of Mayonnaise
- Seasoning

Fats – 35.8g | Protein – 31.2g | Carbs – 12.4g | Calories – 380

To prepare the salad, you can hard boil the egg first. In the meantime, you can prepare the tuna and the avocado which will be sliced. Once the egg is done, you can slice it as well and mix it with the tuna and avocado adding the mayonnaise.

At this point, you can also add the seasoning and any ingredients you might have in the fridge such as a teaspoon of mustard. The mix can also be refrigerated to consume at lunchtime.

Lunch No.7 – Cheeseburger Lettuce Wraps

Cheeseburger lettuce wraps can be prepared easily. This meal can be one of the options to consume either on the spot or refrigerated as needed.

- 2 Pounds Lean Ground Beef With Seasoning
- 6 Slices of Cheddar Cheese
- 2 Large Heads of Iceberg Salad
- 2 Tomatoes
- 1 Large Red Onion

Fats – 18g | Protein – 24g | Carbohydrates – 2g | Calories - 193

To easily prepare this dish you will need to mix the ground beef with your seasoning options. You can now divide the beef into 6 equal pieces to create 6 servings.

They need to be placed in a pan for 4 minutes on each side. When the burgers are done, you will place each one of them on a large piece of lettuce. On top of the burger, you will add a slice of cheese, a slice of

tomato and sliced onion.

Ketogenic Diet Dinner Ideas

Dinner is one of three important meals on the ketogenic diet. But even with no carbs, you can still enjoy a delicious dinner in the comfort of your own home. In order to keep things simple, you will also need to maintain the same minimalistic approach which allows you to stay on target with every dinner, up to 30 days in a row for the length of the diet.

Dinner No.1 – Pork Chops With Asparagus

This simple dinner can be exactly what you need before going to bed as it allows your muscles to recover with complex protein and fats from olive oil. You will need the following ingredients:

- 4oz. Pork Chops
- ½ Cup Of Steamed Asparagus
- 1 Tablespoon of Olive Oil

- 1 Tablespoon of Butter

Fats – 31.7g | Protein – 60g | Carbs – 6.2g | Calories – 317

The pork chops are placed in a nonstick pan with a little olive oil. You will leave them to cook on each side before placing them in the oven. You will leave them in the oven for up to 8 minutes at 140 degrees Fahrenheit. You can now plate the pork chops and add some butter on top of them for extra fats. The asparagus is then added to boiling water. You need to leave it cooking until it reaches tenderness. You will place the asparagus next to the pork chops on the plate when done. With the seasoning you want, this simple recipe can always be a fast solution for a meal which is high in protein and fats. Alternatively, you can reduce the portion of the pork chops if you feel the dinner is too heavy for you.

Dinner No.2 – Salmon with Broccoli

Salmon is one of the most recommended ingredients on the Keto diet and it is easy to understand why. With added cheese and scallions, it can also be one of the meals which are easier on the stomach in the evening.

- 4oz. Salmon
- 1 Tablespoon of Scallions
- 2oz. of Cheddar
- 1 Tablespoon Butter

Fats – 34.6g | Protein – 31.8g | Carbs – 7.8g | Calories – 467

To prepare the salmon you will need to fry it on each side for a few minutes in a pan with butter. The salmon can be prepared in the oven alternatively.

The scallions are finely chopped and placed in a pan with half a tablespoon of butter mixing them lightly to glaze. The grated cheddar is added on top and the mix is removed when the cheese is melted. Plate all ingredients at the end.

Dinner No.3 – Keto Pizza

You are not actually going to eat a real pizza, but you are going to make something which looks like a pizza. Based on eggs, it comes with mozzarella and tomato paste which is close enough when it comes to low carbs.

- 4 Eggs
- 6oz. Shredded Asiago Cheese
- 3 Tablespoons of Tomato Paste
- 1oz. of Pepperoni

Fats – 22.5g | Protein – 15.25g | Carbs – 3.3g | Calories – 274

To prepare the pizza you will need to fry the sliced pepperoni until brown. You will then fry the eggs in a round nonstick pan.

For the next step, you will remove the eggs and place them on a plate. You can add the tomato paste to your liking together with the pepperoni. You need to do this while the eggs are hot because you also need to add the shredded cheese which allows it to melt. There are four servings with each pizza. You can always add a different ingredient to your Keto pizza. An alternative recipe includes added olives or olive oil for a better healthy fats intake.

Dinner No.4 – Steak with Roasted Vegetables

You can never go wrong with a good steak. The best part is that the vegetable options are varied and you can have a different dinner using the same basic approach.

- 1lb Ribeye Steaks
- 1lb Broccoli
- 10oz. Cherry Tomatoes
- 1oz. Anchovies
- 1 Tablespoon of Dried Thyme

Fats – 20.8g | Protein – 28.6g | Carbs – 15g | Calories – 963

To prepare the meal, you can add the vegetables to a large pan and place it in the oven. Keeping it at a temperature of 400 degrees Fahrenheit (200 degrees Celsius) for 15 minutes in the oven is recommended.

The ribeye at room temperature is placed on a frying pan for a few minutes on each side. After 15 minutes, you remove the pan with vegetables from the oven and add the meat. You will then place the tray back into the oven for 10 to 15 minutes. The dinner is one of the most versatile options you can prepare for the Keto diet.

The vegetables can always change and the seasoning can also be different in order to give it a different flavor. You can replace the dried thyme with dried oregano or basil to your taste.

Dinner No.5 – Spicy Thyme Chicken and Coconut Roasted Brussels Sprouts

This healthy dinner can be ready in a short period of time. It combines protein and fats while also being low on carbohydrates. Even more, it also comes with a distinct flavor.

- 1lb Brussels Sprouts
- 2 Chicken Breasts
- 1 Tablespoon Coconut Oil
- 1 Tablespoon Thyme
- ¼ Cup Mustard Lime Dressing

Fats – 16g | Protein – 25g | Carbohydrates – 6g | Calories – 270

To prepare this meal, you will need a large bowl. You will place the sliced chicken breasts into the bowl. Then, you will need to add the mustard and lime dressing together with the thyme.

You need to coat the chicken on all sides and leave to marinate for 15 minutes. In a preheated oven at 350 degrees Fahrenheit, you will add the chicken in a glass baking pan. After 10 minutes, you will add the Brussels sprouts coated with the coconut oil and lightly salted. When you remove the pans from the oven, you can divide the food for two servings.

Dinner No.6 – Shrimp with Tomato and Avocado

This delicious dinner idea can be one of the options to consider when you want a quick meal. Made with scallions and garlic, it is a flavorful dish on the diet.

- 1lbs Shrimp
- 100gr Scallions
- 3 Cloves Garlic
- 1 Avocado

Fats – 14g | Protein – 47.5g | Carbs – 8.5g | Calories – 355

To make the dish you will need to mince the garlic. In a separate bowl, you will season the shrimp with the garlic, salt, pepper, and dried parsley.

The shrimp is placed on a pan and cooked for a minute on each side. Chopped white scallions parts are then added to the pan. In the end, you add the sliced avocado and the chopped green scallions. You can serve the dish like this or with some extra lime squeezed on top. The meal is enough for two portions.

Dinner No.7 – One Pan Chicken with Asparagus

This practical meal can be prepared in 30 minutes and it represents a low-calorie option as each serving comes with 180 calories.

- 4 Pieces of Chicken Breast
- 2 Tablespoons Olive Oil
- 1 Pound Asparagus
- 2 Cloves of Garlic
- 1 Tablespoon of Dijon Mustard
- ½ Lemon Zest

Fats – 14.6g | Protein – 27g | Carbs – 4g | Calories – 180

To prepare the meal you will need to beat down the sliced chicken breast. This allows them to cook evenly. Further, you will need to add them to the pan for 5 minutes on each side. You can then add the olive oil and the asparagus for one minute.

You can now add the garlic and Dijon mustard as well. To finish, you can add the lemon zest and possibly fresh or dried parsley for extra flavor.

Additional Keto Meals

In case you feel that you are still hungry or that you need to adjust some fats or some proteins, you can always have some ingredients ready for meals which can be quickly prepared. These one-pot solutions are convenient and they do not require any advanced cooking skills. Simply dividing the ingredients according to their main nutrients is the best way to go.

Proteins – Eggs, Chicken, Ground Beef, Sausage, and Bacon

Vegetables – Onions, Bell Peppers, Mushrooms, Asparagus, Cherry Tomatoes

Seasoning – Salt, Pepper, Garlic

Fats – Cheeses

These meals are fast to prepare but what about the times when you are away from home? In this case, two options stand out. Healthy snacks based on protein and protein shakes supplements are the best option for a quick caloric intake. Some healthy snacks include jerky or various nuts and seeds. Protein shakes can be easily made with water or coconut water for an extra boost of fats.

30 Day Meal Plan

Included below is a 30 Day Meal Plan featuring all of the meals previously mentioned. Following the plan will give you the best chance for your body to reach a state of Ketosis during the diet. Feel free to mix up the order of the meals to your liking as each meal meets your daily macronutrient allowances.

Day 1

		Fats	Protein	Carbs	Calories
Breakfast	Bulletproof Coffee	18.2	1	0	158
	Fried Eggs with Vegetables and Bacon	30.03	18.7	2.9	320
Lunch	BLT Lettuce Wrap	39	36	3.5	425
Dinner	Pork Chops With Asparagus	31.7	60	6.2	317
	Totals:	119g	116g	13g	1220

Day 2

		Fats	Protein	Carbs	Calories
Breakfast	Bulletproof Coffee	18.2	1	0	158
	Scrambled Eggs	15.5	14.9	0.8	259
Lunch	Beef and Avocado Salad	24.3	19	9	110
Dinner	Salmon with Broccoli	34.6	31.8	7.8	467
	Totals:	93g	67g	18g	994

Day 3

		Fats	Protein	Carbs	Calories
Breakfast	Bulletproof Coffee	18.2	1	0	158
	Cheese with Sausages	31	21	8	393
Lunch	Smoked Salmon with Fresh Spinach	31.6	33.9	3.1	426
Dinner	Keto Pizza	22.5	15.25	3.3	274
	Totals:	103g	71g	14g	1251

Day 4		Fats	Protein	Carbs	Calories
Breakfast	Bulletproof Coffee	18.2	1	0	158
	Cheese Roll-Ups	19.6	6.8	0.4	1020
Lunch	Quesadillas	43.6	14.8	24.5	884
Dinner	Steak with Roasted Vegetables	20.8	28.6	15	963
	Totals:	102g	51g	40g	3025

Day 5		Fats	Protein	Carbs	Calories
Breakfast	BHB Ketones Shake	0	0	0	15
	Fried Eggs with Vegetables and Bacon	30.03	18.7	2.9	320
Lunch	Tuna Avocado Salad	35.8	31.2	12.4	380
Dinner	Spicy Thyme Chicken & Coconut Roasted Brussels	16	25	6	270
	Totals:	82g	75g	21g	985

Day 6		Fats	Protein	Carbs	Calories
Breakfast	Bulletproof Coffee	18.2	1	0	158
	Keto Porridge	62.8	14.3	19.4	712
Lunch	Keto Caesar Salad	28.6	54.8	4	553
Dinner	Shrimp with Tomato and Avocado	14	47.5	8.5	355
	Totals:	124g	118g	32g	1778

Day 7		Fats	Protein	Carbs	Calories
Breakfast	Keto Latte	23.6	6.8	1	278
	Keto Porridge	62.8	14.3	19.4	712
Lunch	Cheeseburger Lettuce Wraps	18	24	2	193
Dinner	One Pan Chicken with Asparagus	14.6	27	4	180
	Totals:	119g	72g	26g	1363

Day 8		Fats	Protein	Carbs	Calories
Breakfast	Bulletproof Coffee	18.2	1	4	158
	Scrambled Eggs	15.5	14.9	0.8	259
Lunch	Beef and Avocado Salad	24.3	19	9	110
Dinner	Salmon with Broccoli	34.6	31.8	7.8	467
	Totals:	93g	67g	22g	994

Day 9		Fats	Protein	Carbs	Calories
Breakfast	Bulletproof Coffee	18.2	1	4	158
	Keto Porridge	62.8	14.3	19.4	712
Lunch	Keto Caesar Salad	28.6	54.8	4	553
Dinner	Shrimp with Tomato and Avocado	14	47.5	8.5	355
	Totals:	124g	118g	36g	1778

Day 10		Fats	Protein	Carbs	Calories
Breakfast	BHB Ketones Shake	0	0	0	15
	Cheese with Sausages	31	21	8	393
Lunch	Tuna Avocado Salad	35.8	31.2	12.4	380
Dinner	Spicy Thyme Chicken & Coconut Roasted Brussels	16	25	6	270
	Totals:	83g	77g	26g	1058

Day 11		Fats	Protein	Carbs	Calories
Breakfast	Keto Latte	23.6	6.8	1	278
	Fried Eggs with Vegetables and Bacon	30.03	18.7	2.9	320
Lunch	BLT Lettuce Wrap	39	36	3.5	425
Dinner	Pork Chops With Asparagus	31.7	60	6.2	317
	Totals:	124g	122g	14g	1340

Day 12		Fats	Protein	Carbs	Calories
Breakfast	Bulletproof Coffee	18.2	1	4	158
	Cheese Roll-Ups	19.6	6.8	0.4	1020
Lunch	Smoked Salmon with Fresh Spinach	31.6	33.9	3.1	426
Dinner	Keto Pizza	22.5	15.25	3.3	274
	Totals:	92g	57g	11g	1878

Day 13		Fats	Protein	Carbs	Calories
Breakfast	Keto Latte	23.6	6.8	1	278
	Scrambled Eggs	15.5	14.9	0.8	259
Lunch	Quesadillas	43.6	14.8	24.5	884
Dinner	Steak with Roasted Vegetables	20.8	28.6	15	963
	Totals:	104g	65g	41g	2384

Day 14		Fats	Protein	Carbs	Calories
Breakfast	Bulletproof Coffee	18.2	1	4	158
	Keto Porridge	62.8	14.3	19.4	712
Lunch	Cheeseburger Lettuce Wraps	18	24	2	193
Dinner	One Pan Chicken with Asparagus	14.6	27	4	180
	Totals:	114g	66g	29g	1243

Day 15		Fats	Protein	Carbs	Calories
Breakfast	Bulletproof Coffee	18.2	1	4	158
	Fried Eggs with Vegetables and Bacon	30.03	18.7	2.9	320
Lunch	BLT Lettuce Wrap	39	36	3.5	425
Dinner	Pork Chops With Asparagus	31.7	60	6.2	317
	Totals:	119g	116g	17g	1220

Day 16		Fats	Protein	Carbs	Calories
Breakfast	Bulletproof Coffee	18.2	1	4	158
	Cheese Roll-Ups	19.6	6.8	0.4	1020
Lunch	Quesadillas	43.6	14.8	24.5	884
Dinner	Steak with Roasted Vegetables	20.8	28.6	15	963
	Totals:	102g	51g	44g	3025

Day 17		Fats	Protein	Carbs	Calories
Breakfast	BHB Ketones Shake	0	0	0	15
	Scrambled Eggs	15.5	14.9	0.8	259
Lunch	Beef and Avocado Salad	24.3	19	9	110
Dinner	Salmon with Broccoli	34.6	31.8	7.8	467
	Totals:	74g	66g	18g	851

Day 18		Fats	Protein	Carbs	Calories
Breakfast	Keto Latte	23.6	6.8	1	278
	Cheese with Sausages	31	21	8	393
Lunch	Smoked Salmon with Fresh Spinach	31.6	33.9	3.1	426
Dinner	Keto Pizza	22.5	15.25	3.3	274
	Totals:	109g	77g	15g	1371

Day 19		Fats	Protein	Carbs	Calories
Breakfast	Bulletproof Coffee	18.2	1	4	158
	Keto Porridge	62.8	14.3	19.4	712
Lunch	Keto Caesar Salad	28.6	54.8	4	553
Dinner	Shrimp with Tomato and Avocado	14	47.5	8.5	355
	Totals:	124g	118g	36g	1778

Day 20		Fats	Protein	Carbs	Calories
Breakfast	Bulletproof Coffee	18.2	1	4	158
	Scrambled Eggs	15.5	14.9	0.8	259
Lunch	Cheeseburger Lettuce Wraps	18	24	2	193
Dinner	One Pan Chicken with Asparagus	14.6	27	4	180
	Totals:	66g	67g	11g	790

Day 21		Fats	Protein	Carbs	Calories
Breakfast	Keto Latte	23.6	6.8	1	278
	Scrambled Eggs	15.5	14.9	0.8	259
Lunch	Beef and Avocado Salad	24.3	19	9	110
Dinner	Steak with Roasted Vegetables	20.8	28.6	15	963
	Totals:	84g	69g	26g	1610

Day 22		Fats	Protein	Carbs	Calories
Breakfast	BHB Ketones Shake	0	0	0	15
	Cheese with Sausages	31	21	8	393
Lunch	Smoked Salmon with Fresh Spinach	31.6	33.9	3.1	426
Dinner	Shrimp with Tomato and Avocado	14	47.5	8.5	355
	Totals:	77g	102g	20g	1189

Day 23		Fats	Protein	Carbs	Calories
Breakfast	Bulletproof Coffee	18.2	1	4	158
	Cheese Roll-Ups	31	21	8	393
Lunch	Quesadillas	43.6	14.8	24.5	884
Dinner	Keto Pizza	22.5	15.25	3.3	274
	Totals:	115g	52g	40g	1709

Day 24		Fats	Protein	Carbs	Calories
Breakfast	Bulletproof Coffee	18.2	1	4	158
	Fried Eggs with Vegetables and Bacon	30.03	18.7	2.9	320
Lunch	Cheeseburger Lettuce Wraps	18	24	2	193
Dinner	Pork Chops With Asparagus	31.7	60	6.2	317
	Totals:	98g	104g	15g	988

Day 25		Fats	Protein	Carbs	Calories
Breakfast	Bulletproof Coffee	18.2	1	4	158
	Keto Porridge	62.8	14.3	19.4	712
Lunch	Tuna Avocado Salad	35.8	31.2	12.4	380
Dinner	Spicy Thyme Chicken & Coconut Roasted Brussels	16	25	6	270
	Totals:	133g	72g	42g	1520

Day 26		Fats	Protein	Carbs	Calories
Breakfast	Bulletproof Coffee	18.2	1	4	158
	Cheese with Sausages	31	21	8	393
Lunch	BLT Lettuce Wrap	39	36	3.5	425
Dinner	Salmon with Broccoli	34.6	31.8	7.8	467
	Totals:	123g	90g	23g	1443

Day 27		Fats	Protein	Carbs	Calories
Breakfast	Bulletproof Coffee	18.2	1	4	158
	Scrambled Eggs	15.5	14.9	0.8	259
Lunch	Keto Caesar Salad	28.6	54.8	4	553
Dinner	One Pan Chicken with Asparagus	14.6	27	4	180
	Totals:	77g	98g	13g	1150

<u>**Day 28**</u>

		Fats	**Protein**	**Carbs**	**Calories**
Breakfast	Bulletproof Coffee	18.2	1	4	158
	Fried Eggs with Vegetables and Bacon	30.03	18.7	2.9	320
Lunch	Smoked Salmon with Fresh Spinach	31.6	33.9	3.1	426
Dinner	Keto Pizza	22.5	15.25	3.3	274
	Totals:	102g	69g	13g	1178

<u>**Day 29**</u>

		Fats	**Protein**	**Carbs**	**Calories**
Breakfast	Keto Latte	23.6	6.8	1	278
	Cheese Roll-Ups	19.6	6.8	0.4	1020
Lunch	Beef and Avocado Salad	24.3	19	9	110
Dinner	Steak with Roasted Vegetables	20.8	28.6	15	963
	Totals:	88g	61g	25g	2371

<u>**Day 30**</u>

		Fats	**Protein**	**Carbs**	**Calories**
Breakfast	Bulletproof Coffee	18.2	1	4	158
	Scrambled Eggs	15.5	14.9	0.8	259
Lunch	Tuna Avocado Salad	35.8	31.2	12.4	380
Dinner	One Pan Chicken with Asparagus	14.6	27	4	180
	Totals:	84g	74g	21g	977

Chapter 5: Counting Calories

Ketosis and calories go hand in hand. But there are many questions which are often addressed to the benefits of the Keto diet in regards to a calorie surplus. It is therefore worth addressing this question and other calorie questions before you actually start to diet.

Is Ketosis Possible With Increased Calories?

As one of the main questions with ketosis, this needs to be addressed from the start. Can you lose weight actually eating more calories, even if they are healthy calories?

In theory, the one thing which matters most is calories in versus calories out. In other words, the number of consumed calories is what dictates weight loss. But at the same time, the quality of the calories is also very important. In a simple example, you can imagine consuming fewer calories only from sugar and carbohydrates and what they can do to your fitness level. This is why most diets actually reduce and eliminate bad calories. Before actually basing their approach on the number of calories to be consumed, most diets recommend eating healthier foods. This is also the case of the Ketogenic diet as well.

Another interesting aspect of the high fat and low sugar diets is that they regularly offer people the choice of how much food they can actually consume. Since fats are so satiating, you do not feel the need to consume as many calories as with other diets. In other words, overeating is not as common on the Keto diet as on other diets which are not as high in fats.

Another aspect to remember is that the needed calories for an average adult can also vary daily. This is why all the recommendations are actually made on averages. In most cases, even hormonal activity such as cortisol, testosterone or estrogen can impact the calories needed every day. So while in theory caloric deficit is required to lose weight, it is hard to establish what this deficit really means if you want to quantify it.

But since there are different types of calories, you need to know that there are different types of fats as well. The human body has brown fat and white fat. Brown fat comes with the role of keeping you warm. Thus, the calories you consume for this type of fat are actual calories you consume just to keep you warm. This type of fat is not used for energy. It has a thermogenic role and it is burned for heat. White fat is burnt for ATP (intracellular energy) and it is what the Keto diet is based on.

Putting these theories into practice, you can be in the state of ketosis. At this point, you decide to consume some fats such as MCT oil. This is going to act as a catalyst for your ketosis. So consuming different calories comes with different results. 1 gram of sugar can trigger insulin and open the doors for fat storage while one gram of fat can be used for energy. This is why the number of calories always matters but their quality matters as well.

How to Avoid Caloric Mistakes?

When it comes to the success of the Keto diet, it all has to do with the number of fats you consume. A lot of data we have on the effects of ketosis are actually based on more radical approaches to the Keto diet which can be the case with up to 90% fat consumption. Mainly used in various therapies, this radical approach is not sustainable for most people.

But still, you need to know that around 75% of your actual calories need to come from fats.

Consume Enough Fats

The biggest mistake people make while on the Keto diet is simply not consuming enough fats, therefore, their diet becomes strongly based on protein. When people don't see any results they often try to increase fats but they maintain that same approach with protein and this is why they might even be consuming more calories than what is required. In most situations, it is also true that many people simply do not know what to expect in terms of calories. Making a pizza with a chicken breast crust is not the best option for high fat intake. The keto diet is characterized by moderate protein intake and your number one ingredient still needs to be fat.

Measure Ketone Levels

The days of guessing on the Keto diet are long gone. There are many options which now allow you to measure your ketone levels. Ketone test strips are affordable and they can be found easily in many health stores. This is why you now have the ability to know your ketone levels every day and this allows you to tweak your foods accordingly. Keto strips measure acetate in urine.

Alternative methods involve taking blood samples. This specific method is one of the most reliable options to measure ketone levels and it can indicate your level of ketosis. The tests measure BHB levels.

Another method can involve using your smartphone. A breath acetone analyzer is one of the most practical methods of measuring your ketosis. The main advantage of this option comes with the archiving possibilities on your smartphone. You are able to check your progress on your smartphone and see how your acetone levels changed from Week 1 to Week 4.

Drink Plenty of Water

Water is crucial during the Ketogenic diet. Factual data shows that for every 3.7g of carbohydrates consumed, you hold 4 grams of water. Depriving your body of carbs can cause water loss. This means that you can even become dehydrated on the diet. Furthermore, insulin levels are also low on the diet since insulin tells your kidneys when to retain water and when to flush it, ketosis could cause unbalanced hydration levels.

The fact that the body retains water with carbs is not a major concern. However, since the kidneys will not signal for the hydration required by the body means that you need to drink plenty of water. In the case of the ketogenic diet, you will actually see water going through the system quickly so expect plenty of visits to the restroom.

Take Minerals Seriously

Consuming enough minerals is crucial in the situation in which you urinate a lot. This is where magnesium, sodium, and potassium are often low on the Keto diet. Some of the steps you can apply to ensure that this is not your case is to simply use plenty of salt with each meal. You can also consume foods which are rich in minerals such as spinach or almonds. At the same time, you should also consider a good supplement if you cannot meet the daily needs for minerals.

Calories from Alcohol and Dehydration

Fatty acid oxidant and ketone production occur in the liver but alcohol consumption prevents this from happening. In other words, the more you drink the less able your liver will be able to produce ketones. The whole principle of the diet is to have high fatty acids in the bloodstream but alcohol stops this from happening. This means that you will not be able to see the benefits you want when it comes to overall weight loss. Even more, you will see a detrimental effect on your health as in the absence of glucose and of ketones from the blood; your body will enter a state of starvation.

In simple terms of calories, you want to avoid beer. 100 grams of beer can come with 43 calories and 3.6 grams of carbohydrates. If you have to drink, spirits might be a better option even when compared to wine. But generally speaking, you want to avoid alcohol for the duration of the diet and limit it in general if you want to maintain a healthy weight.

Caloric Tips for Faster Ketosis

Entering ketosis faster is the key to its success. Consuming the right calories is crucial when you want to maintain it. Here are a few tips you can apply when it comes to reaching this fat-burning state.

Consume Caffeine

A study showed that people who consumed high levels of caffeine had nearly double the number of ketones in their blood. Consuming plenty of black coffee is one of the main drivers of ketone increase.

Caffeine is also going to help your body with its metabolism. Drinking plenty of coffee acts as a catalyst and helps the conversion of fats into ketones.

MCT Oil

With a similar effect but with a direct source of fatty acids, MCT oil is directly absorbed into the bloodstream from digestion. Bypassing the liver, MCT's are utilized directly for ketone production. The good news is that MCT oil can be consumed as needed throughout the diet.

Fasting

If you are starting to see that you are getting out of ketosis before Week 4, you can always rely on fasting to get back on track. If you are fasting, your body will start to produce ketones in the absence of glucose from your bloodstream. At the same time, if you are already in a state of ketosis and you want to further improve your results, fasting can be one of the proven ways to essentially mobilize more ketones which can be immediately used for energy.

Fasting also has a range of benefits which go beyond ketones. It can also help you improve cognition and neuron communication. This makes one of the natural ways of improving your mental focus capacity. In the long-term, it can be used as a trigger to boost fat loss efforts as well so adapting to fasting can be beneficial even when your diet is completed.

Chapter 6: Maintaining the Results of the Diet

One of the major issues with the Keto diet or any other diet comes with the sustainability of the results. Most studies show that this is where many people tend to bounce back to the weight they had before the diet. In many cases, this is simply due to reversing your lifestyle back to what it used to be. Therefore, when you are in Week 4 of the Keto diet, you need to think of more permanent solutions to allow your body to naturally burn fat and stay fit for longer. This doesn't mean that you cannot consume carbohydrates again, but it means that you need to know how to use food and exercise to your advantage.

Long-Term Diets

While you can always come back to the Keto diet to lose more weight, it is also recommended maintaining a lower body fat percentage which makes the task of the diet easier in the future as well. Generally speaking, you need to consume foods which are healthy for the most part. Of course, you can indulge in the occasional cakes, but it is what you consume most that influences your body weight.

One thing you can apply to your nutrition from the Keto diet comes with fats consumption. Eat healthy fats in the long-term and you can reap visible benefits. While you will not consume as many fats as on the diet, you can still add avocados, macadamia nuts, and coconut oil to your foods from time to time. While supplements are also available, it is also recommended to look for the options which allow you to consume these fats in your diet.

Omega 3 fats are important for your health. You can source them from different types of seafood and fish. With an important role in fat burning, they are also important when it comes to joint health as well. One of the most qualitative sources of fats comes from Krill oil. Similar to fish oil, Krill oil also comes with Astaxanthin which is a powerful antioxidant and is not found in regular fish oil. With an important impact reducing oxidative stress, the oil can be consumed from time to time as an alternative to the more affordable supplements with fatty acids.

Caloric Quality and Quantity

Another important element comes with the quality of the calories you consume after the diet. This is why it is important to look for the options which are sustainable for the long-term, which is not the case with the foods of the Keto diet. So what can you consume?

You should always aim to consume foods which are not highly processed. The more processed the foods, the less available they are in nutrients for your overall health not only for weight loss. In order to simplify your approach, dividing your nutrients similarly to the classification found on the Keto diet can make the process simpler. You can divide your foods by macronutrients and micronutrients as follows:

- Carbohydrates – A Source Of Energy
- Fats – A Soluble Source Of Energy
- Fiber – Indigestible Portion With A Role In The Health Of The Digestive System
- Proteins – Essential For Muscle Repair And Growth

- Minerals – Inorganic Elements Essential For The Body
- Vitamins – Essential Role In The Chemical Processes Of The Body

Carbohydrates can be consumed after the diet but you will benefit the most simply by choosing healthier options instead of the processed carbs. Foods such as oatmeal, brown rice or sweet potatoes are essential for your health and even for some brain processes. If you think that carbs will make you gain weight again, a simple way to consume them is immediately after a workout when your muscles need them the most. Other carbs such as oats are also consumed before workouts for better energy.

Fats are essential even outside the Ketogenic diet. A good source of Omega 3 or healthy fats such as those from coconut oil is recommended for most people as they can help the regulation of hormones.

But the fats from meats are not the only options to consider. Fats from nuts and seeds are also highly recommended. Unsaturated and monounsaturated fats from nuts are a good source of amino acids. This is why a balanced diet which is based on fats from meats, fish and vegan alternatives is always recommended.

Fiber is essential for the health of the digestive system and also for the health of your intestines. Eating more vegetables and grains is highly recommended. Green leafy vegetables can be a good source of fiber and they can also come with added minerals as well.

Even when you are not on the Keto diet, protein plays an important role. This is where you want to ensure that you are capable to deliver great results when it comes to better overall health, especially the health of the muscles and of the joints. Investing in high-quality protein such as grass-fed beef, milk, eggs or fish is always recommended. You can also experiment some of the vegan proteins even if you eat meat for better nutrient variation. This means that you can source these proteins from nuts or you can even find some delicious alternatives such as a peanut butter with no sugar.

Minerals are also required for good health. They can be found in most foods. Vegetable and fruit consumption is recommended when you want to have the best overall results, especially for a balanced diet every day. Many health organizations recommend at least 5 fruits and vegetables to be consumed every day.

Vitamins are not as easy to find in supplements. But in fruits and vegetables, they come with their natural nutrition value which is not made in a lab meaning that they can be used by the body. However, you cannot consume these foods sporadically to boost vitamin intake if you want the best health. You need to consume them extensively in order to be able to gather all their benefits. Natural juices are not the best alternative though as they can come with no fiber or with a higher sugar content, which is not healthy either.

Great Hydration

Hydration always needs to be on point if you want to have a healthy weight. A simple rule is to simply avoid being thirsty as you should always be hydrating yourself. Hydration means plain water not juices, sodas or other fizzy drinks. Your body needs fresh water to run at an optimum level.

In many cases, people are dramatically dehydrated. This is why it is recommended to always have water with you when needed and this gives you the freedom to maintain hydration levels even away from home.

Exercise Routines

Exercise plays a crucial role in the overall health and even in the weight management process. If you cannot play a sport, you can simply start to take long walks. If you can play a sport, enjoying more active time outdoors can be highly recommended and it can keep certain cardiovascular problems away.

Even joining a gym is recommended when compared to an inactive lifestyle. You can combine strength training with cardiovascular training to allow for great results when it comes to maintaining that lower body fat percentage. There are various recent studies which show that muscles are efficient at burning fat so when you improve your strength and muscle size, your body will be better at burning fat.

As one of the most recommended solutions to maintain the post-Keto results, it can also be a solution to keep cholesterol levels low. But exercising also has multiple benefits on the brain and mood. This is why it is highly advised to consider more physical activity if you are fighting issues such as depression or anxiety as well. In many cases, these issues can keep you away from making healthier lifestyle choices.

When considering lifestyle choices, fast-foods, alcohol, and smoking need to be controlled or even eliminated. Packed with calories, fast-foods are a rapid source of weight gain. Alcohol can also be detrimental to your health and it can lead to weight gain and especially fat gains around the waist which has been linked to possible cardiovascular problems. Smoking negatively impacts your health at multiple levels as well. Make sure that your 4-week effort on the Keto diet was not in vain and try to minimize these vices going forward.

Proper Resting

Resting time is essential for recovery. Your muscles and your brain need proper rest every night. This also allows your hormones to stay in balance and this is why it is so important to find the right schedule which allows you not to stay up late and to actually get rested every night. You want to avoid the overuse of coffee or other stimulants for energy and you need to listen to your body when it's signaling to you that it needs to rest.

Proper rest is difficult to establish so in order to be well-rested all of the time; you need to establish a clear routine which allows you to go to bed when you need to. Studies also find that a single night of proper rest per week can get you back on track for previous nights in which you didn't get enough rest. So this recovery process can be seen both with muscle recovery and better mood as well. It is also recommended to adjust your sleeping time so that you get an uninterrupted resting interval within specific hours. Research shows that a colder room is preferred to a hotter room when it comes to good rest.

Fasting

If you want to experience something closer to the Keto diet but not an actual diet in itself, fasting can represent a great way to control body fat. There are different types of fasting which you can follow. One of the most popular types of fasting over recent years comes with intermittent fasting. This allows you to consume calories only in a certain timeframe during the day.

For example, you can decide to consume foods only after 11 AM and together with the hours of the night, it can lead to a fasting period of more than 12 hours. This can allow you to optimize fat loss and this is why it is also used by fitness people who are looking to minimize their body fat percentage.

This approach is also less drastic than committing to a full day of fasting. It allows you to concentrate on the best results when it comes to sustainability as well. At the same time, you do not need to exclude any type of nutrients in the feeding window.

For the best results with your new lower weight after the Keto diet, the combination of healthy foods, proper hydration, an exercise routine and plenty of resting time is essential. This is why you need to know that you can experience weight loss naturally which is also one of the principles of the Keto diet. In short, there are a few characteristics of the diet which can be used in the future as well:

- Nutrient Quality
- Healthy Fats Consumption
- Protein Consumption For Muscle Repair
- Possible Fasting For Enhanced Fat Burning

Conclusion

It is highly recommended to look at the Ketogenic diet from a planned perspective. As outlined before, the diet started nearly a century ago under medical supervision for totally different reasons and this is why you need to expect some other health benefits in the area of cognition as well.

However, the main purpose of the Keto diet is to bring you into the state of ketosis which uses ketones instead of glucose for energy. With the 4-week food and supplements plan, you can draw out exactly the breakfasts, lunches and dinners you are going to consume.

As a summary, your first days on the diet will also be the hardest. You can experience the Keto flu issue during these days. The best way to tackle it is to start consuming fats to have an energy source in your body which allows you to minimize this potential issue. If you want quicker results, fasting can also be recommended. Even the first day of Week 1 can be started with the Keto *Bulletproof coffee* which is a combination of regular black coffee and MCT oil. It allows you a good overall energy boost and it can help the transition towards ketosis as well. Furthermore, it is also recommended to look at the foods which, at the end of the day, need to be around the 75% fats, 20% protein and 5% carbs ratio. The closer you are to this, the better. If you are unsure, you always need to increase fat consumption as it is largely responsible for satiety and it will keep you on track with controlling cravings as well.

The Keto diet is also largely different to what it was in the early 1900s. You do not have to wait weeks to see if you lose weight or even if you are in the state of ketosis. You can use one of the outlined testing methods to establish your ketone levels on the spot.

At the same time, modern Keto diets benefit from supplements which were not available decades ago. This includes pure MCT oil, pre-workouts with MCT's, protein powders with MCTs, BHB supplements for instant exogenous ketones or even greens for complete micronutrient content. In most cases, you also need to follow the solutions which allow you to add quality to your diet as you can also find most of these ingredients in foods. Supplementation can prove to be an asset when it comes to reaching ketosis faster. In most cases, it is only recommended to use high-quality products based on fats from foods such as coconuts, macadamia nuts, whey or pea protein.

Successfully navigating from Week 1 to Week 4 is based on planning. You can prepare the mentioned meals with a minimum list of ingredients to make this period simpler. At the same time, you can complete your daily nutrition with supplements. As mentioned before, drinking more water is strongly advised as well. The low carbohydrate diet is strongly based on the fats and this is why you always need to prioritize them before protein.

In most cases, you also need to reintroduce carbohydrates into your diet gradually. The week following the diet is a transition period in which you start to consume small amounts of carbs again. At the same time, it is also the week to start applying recommended advice when it comes to keeping your weight as you don't want to be one of the people who gain all the weight back after the diet.

Finally, if you enjoyed this book, please take the time to share your thoughts and post a review on Amazon. It would be greatly appreciated!